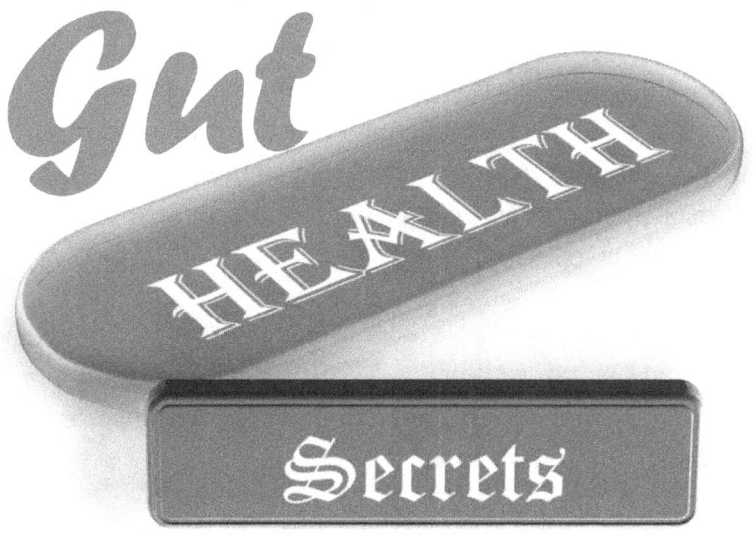

Gut HEALTH Secrets

100 Powerful Solutions to Transform Your Gut
Microbiome and Enhance Your health

By

Bailey Kingsford

I dedicate this book to all those seeking vibrant health and a renewed sense of well-being. May it serve as a guiding light on your journey toward optimal gut health and inspire you to unlock the secrets within.

Disclaimer: The information provided in this book is for educational purposes only and is not intended as a substitute for professional medical advice, diagnosis, or treatment. Always seek the advice of your physician or other qualified health provider with any questions you may have regarding a medical condition or before embarking on any new health regimen.

TABLE OF CONTENTS

Introduction

Unlock the Secrets to Vibrant Health with "Gut Health Secrets: Transform Your Gut Microbiome with 100 Powerful Solutions for Enhanced Health." Are you tired of feeling sluggish, bloated, and lacking energy? Do you long for a revitalized body and mind? Look no further – this groundbreaking guide is your ticket to a transformative journey toward optimal well-being.

Inside the pages of "Gut Health Secrets," you'll embark on an empowering quest to revolutionize your gut microbiome. Prepare to be captivated as you delve into the hidden realm of your gut, discovering its profound influence on your overall health. It's time to break free from the chains of digestive discomfort and unleash a new, vibrant you.

Imagine a life where you no longer suffer from bloating, irregular bowel movements, or constant fatigue. Picture yourself experiencing a deep sense of vitality, mental clarity, and emotional stability.

With the expert strategies and insights shared within this book, you'll be equipped with 100 powerful solutions to reclaim control over your gut health.

Get ready to embark on a life-changing journey as you unlock the secrets of your gut and unveil a path to enhanced health and wellness.

Embrace the opportunity to transform your life from the inside out and discover the true potential that lies within you. Your vibrant future awaits, and "Gut Health Secrets" is your guiding light on this extraordinary quest.

Chapter one

Unveiling Your Gut Issues: Tests, Analysis, and Insights for Restoring Gut Health

Are you tired of feeling trapped in a cycle of discomfort and confusion? Your gut health might hold the key to unlocking a vibrant and energized life. Imagine bidding farewell to the persistent bloating, unpredictable bowel movements, and relentless fatigue. It's time to embark on a journey of self-discovery, understanding, and healing.

When it comes to unraveling the mysteries of your gut, comprehensive tests are essential. From stool analyses to food sensitivity panels, these tests provide a window into your body's inner workings.

They help identify hidden culprits that sabotage your well-being, allowing you to reclaim control over your health. As you receive the results, a whirlwind of emotions may wash over you—relief, curiosity, and perhaps a pinch of anxiety. Embrace it all, for knowledge is power.

The analysis phase is where the puzzle pieces start falling into place. Skilled practitioners will guide you through the intricate details, explaining how each finding correlates to your symptoms.

Aha moments become frequent visitors, connecting the dots and revealing the intricate dance between your gut and overall health. Embrace this process of discovery, for it is an investment in your future.

Insights gained from these tests are the guiding stars that illuminate your path towards restoring gut health. Armed with knowledge, you'll embark on a personalized healing journey.

A journey that may involve dietary adjustments, targeted supplementation, stress management, and the integration of mindful practices. Along the way, you'll witness your body's incredible resilience and capacity for transformation.

It won't be a linear journey; there will be setbacks and challenges. Yet, armed with newfound insights, you'll have the tools to navigate through them. As you progress, you'll start noticing the subtle shifts—a surge of energy, a calm gut, and a sense of well-being that permeates your being.

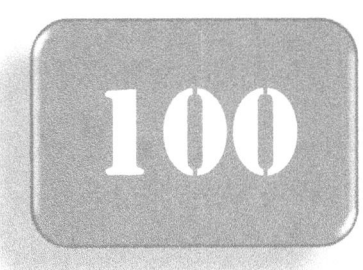

100

Powerful Solutions
to
Transform Your

Gut Microbiome

Develop a morning routine

Establishing a consistent morning routine can positively affect your gut microbiome and set a healthy tone for the day. Start by waking up at a regular time, allowing yourself enough sleep for adequate rest and recovery.

Incorporate activities such as;

- Mindfulness meditation,
- Stretching or yoga, and
- A balanced breakfast.
- Hydrate with a glass of water, as proper hydration supports digestion and nutrient absorption.
- Taking time for self-care and planning the day ahead can reduce stress and contribute to better gut health.

Release your thoughts through a brain dump

Engaging in a brain dump exercise can help reduce mental clutter, stress, and indirectly support your gut microbiome. A brain dump involves writing down all your thoughts, worries, or to-do lists onto paper or a digital document.

By externalizing your thoughts, you can declutter your mind, alleviate stress, and create space for more positive and focused thinking. Set aside dedicated time for a brain dump exercise, preferably in a quiet and comfortable environment. Let your thoughts flow freely without judgment, allowing for mental and emotional release.

#3

Retreat to nature

Spending time in nature can have a profound impact on your gut microbiome and overall health. Studies suggest that exposure to natural environments can increase microbial diversity, boost immune function, and reduce stress levels.

Take regular breaks to immerse yourself in nature, whether it's walking in a park, hiking in the woods, or simply sitting by a lake or beach. Engage your senses by observing the sights, listening to the sounds, and connecting with the natural world around you.

#4

Smile at yourself in the mirror

Practicing self-affirmation and self-love can positively influence your gut microbiome. Smiling at yourself in the mirror is a simple yet powerful way to cultivate self-compassion and boost mood.

When you smile, your body releases endorphins, which can reduce stress and promote overall well-being. Spend a few moments each day smiling at yourself in the mirror, appreciating your unique qualities, and reaffirming positive affirmations. This practice can shift your mindset, increase self-esteem, and indirectly benefit your gut health.

Select your thoughts consciously

Being mindful of your thoughts and consciously choosing positive and constructive thinking patterns can transform your gut microbiome. Negative thought patterns, such as rumination or self-criticism, can increase stress levels and affect gut health.

Practice awareness of your thoughts and challenge negative or unhelpful thinking. Cultivate positive affirmations, gratitude, and self-compassion.

Engage in mindfulness or meditation practices to cultivate a more positive and balanced mindset. By consciously selecting your thoughts, you can foster a healthier gut microbiome and overall well-being.

Alter your "what-if" scenarios

Constantly engaging in "what-if" scenarios and catastrophic thinking can contribute to stress and negatively impact your gut microbiome. Instead, strive to alter these thought patterns and focus on realistic and positive alternatives.

When negative "what-if" thoughts arise, consciously shift your focus to more constructive possibilities. Practice grounding techniques, deep breathing exercises, or redirect your attention to the present moment.

By altering your "what-if" scenarios, you can reduce stress levels and create a more positive mental environment that supports gut health.

Schedule worry time

Rather than allowing worries to consume your entire day, allocate specific time for focused worry. By scheduling worry time, you can contain your worries and prevent them from overwhelming your thoughts throughout the day.

Choose a consistent time slot, preferably earlier in the day, and dedicate 10-15 minutes to consciously exploring your worries. Write them down, reflect on possible solutions or alternative perspectives, and make a conscious effort to release them outside of the designated worry time.

This practice can reduce stress and prevent prolonged exposure to negative thinking patterns that affect gut health.

Delegate tasks

Taking on too much responsibility can lead to chronic stress and negatively impact your gut microbiome. Learning to delegate tasks and ask for help when needed is crucial for maintaining a healthy balance.

Assess your commitments and responsibilities, identify tasks that can be delegated to others, and communicate your needs effectively.

Delegate tasks at work, involve family members in household chores, or seek assistance from friends or professionals. By sharing the load, you can reduce stress, create more time for self-care, and support your gut health.

#9

Establish boundaries

Setting healthy boundaries is essential for maintaining a positive gut microbiome. Boundaries protect your physical and mental well-being, preventing stress and negative influences from disrupting gut health.

Clearly communicate your limits and expectations to others, learn to say no when necessary, and prioritize self-care. Evaluate your relationships and environments, reducing exposure to toxic or draining situations.

By establishing and maintaining boundaries, you create a supportive environment that fosters better gut health and overall well-being.

#10

Validate yourself and your accomplishments

Acknowledging and celebrating your achievements is essential for nurturing a positive mindset and indirectly improving your gut microbiome. Self-validation enhances self-esteem, reduces stress, and fosters a sense of self-worth.

Regularly reflect on your accomplishments, both big and small, and give yourself credit for your efforts and achievements. Practice positive self-talk and embrace self-compassion.

Engage in activities that make you feel accomplished and proud, and surround yourself with supportive individuals who recognize and validate your growth and achievements.

#11

Focus on how you can help others

Shifting your focus from self-centered thoughts to helping others can positively impact your gut microbiome. Engaging in acts of kindness and empathy promotes a sense of purpose, fulfillment, and overall well-being.

Volunteer your time, lend a helping hand to someone in need, or participate in community initiatives. By focusing on how you can make a positive difference in the lives of others, you cultivate a sense of connection, reduce stress, and indirectly support your gut health.

Remember, even small acts of kindness can have a significant impact on your well-being and the well-being of others.

Confront your fears head-on

Confronting your fears directly can be a powerful way to improve your gut microbiome and overall health. Fear and anxiety trigger stress responses in the body, which can disrupt the balance of gut bacteria.

Identify your fears and break them down into manageable steps. Gradually expose yourself to the things that make you anxious, challenging yourself to face them head-on.

Seek support from a therapist or counselor if needed. By confronting your fears, you can reduce anxiety, increase resilience, and support a healthier gut microbiome.

Relax and unwind

Engaging in regular relaxation practices is essential for promoting a healthy gut microbiome. Chronic stress negatively affects gut health, so it's crucial to counterbalance it with relaxation techniques.

Find activities that help you unwind and destress, such as;

- Practicing yoga
- Taking nature walks
- Listening to calming music, or
- Practicing deep breathing exercises.

Make time for relaxation each day, even if it's just a few minutes. Prioritize self-care and create a calm and peaceful space where you can truly relax and rejuvenate.

#14

Request assistance when needed

Asking for help when you need it is a vital aspect of maintaining a healthy gut microbiome and overall well-being. Trying to do everything on your own can lead to overwhelm and increased stress levels.

Recognize your limitations and reach out to others for support. Whether it's seeking guidance from a healthcare professional, delegating tasks to colleagues or family members, or seeking emotional support from friends, don't hesitate to ask for assistance.

By seeking help, you can alleviate stress, lighten your load, and create a more balanced and supportive environment for your gut health to thrive.

#15

Say farewell to plastic

Plastic is known to release harmful chemicals that can disrupt the balance of your gut microbiome and have adverse effects on your health. By reducing your plastic consumption, you can minimize your exposure to these toxins and support a healthier gut.

Start by;

- Replacing single-use plastic items such as water bottles, food containers, and utensils with reusable alternatives made from glass, stainless steel, or BPA-free materials.
- Use eco-friendly cloth bags for shopping and opt for fresh produce without plastic packaging whenever possible.

Additionally, support initiatives that promote plastic waste reduction and recycling to contribute to a healthier environment and gut microbiome.

#16

Drink water immediately upon waking up

Drinking water first thing in the morning can have a positive impact on your gut microbiome and overall health. It helps to rehydrate your body after hours of sleep and kick-start your digestive system.

Drinking water in the morning can stimulate bowel movements, support the elimination of waste, and promote a healthy gut environment.

To achieve this habit;

- keep a glass or bottle of water by your bedside and make it a priority to drink it as soon as you wake up.
- Aim for at least 8 ounces (240 ml) of water to replenish your body and optimize your gut health.

Heat your water before consuming

Consuming warm water, especially before meals, can aid digestion and promote a healthier gut microbiome. Warm water helps to stimulate the production of digestive enzymes, improves blood circulation to the gut, and enhances nutrient absorption.

To incorporate this practice into your routine;

- Heat a cup of water to a comfortable temperature (not boiling) and drink it around 15-30 minutes before meals.

This habit can support better digestion, nutrient absorption, and a balanced gut microbiome.

#18

Avoid burning scented candles

Scented candles often contain synthetic fragrances and chemicals that can disrupt the balance of your gut microbiome and negatively impact your health.

These chemicals can contribute to inflammation and reduce the diversity of beneficial gut bacteria. Instead of burning scented candles, opt for natural alternatives such as beeswax or soy candles, which emit fewer harmful compounds.

Alternatively, consider using essential oil diffusers or natural room sprays to create a pleasant atmosphere without compromising your gut health.

#19

Avoid eating snacks late at night

Late-night snacking can disrupt your circadian rhythm and negatively affect your gut microbiome. Your gut follows a natural rhythm that aligns with your sleep-wake cycle, and eating late can disrupt this balance.

When you eat late at night, your digestive system has to work harder, potentially leading to indigestion, disrupted sleep, and imbalanced gut bacteria.

To support a healthy gut;

- Aim to finish your last meal or snack at least two to three hours before bedtime.

This allows your digestive system to rest and recover during the night, promoting a more balanced gut microbiome.

Sleep on the left side of your body

The position in which you sleep can impact your gut health. Sleeping on your left side has been found to have potential benefits for digestion and gut microbiome balance. This position can help facilitate the proper flow of waste and toxins through your digestive system.

When you sleep on your left side, gravity aids in the movement of food waste from the small intestine to the large intestine, promoting regular bowel movements and reducing the likelihood of constipation.

To adopt this position;

- Try using a body pillow or adjust your sleeping position gradually until you find comfort on your left side.

Scrape your tongue for oral hygiene

Tongue scraping is an effective practice for oral hygiene that can also positively influence your gut microbiome. Your tongue harbors bacteria, debris, and toxins that can contribute to an imbalanced gut environment when swallowed. By regularly scraping your tongue, you remove these harmful substances and promote oral health.

To scrape your tongue;

- Use a tongue scraper (available in pharmacies or online) and gently scrape from the back of your tongue to the front.
- Rinse the scraper between each scrape, and repeat the process a few times.

Incorporate this practice into your daily oral hygiene routine to maintain a healthy oral microbiome and support a balanced gut.

Wake up and take a walk

Engaging in physical activity, such as taking a walk, in the morning can have positive effects on your gut microbiome and overall health. Morning exercise helps stimulate bowel movements, supporting regularity and optimal gut function.

It can also reduce stress levels, which can directly impact the diversity and health of your gut bacteria.

To achieve this;

- Set aside time in the morning for a brisk walk or light exercise.
- Start with a few minutes and gradually increase the duration and intensity.

Remember to listen to your body and choose activities that you enjoy to make it a sustainable habit.

Establish a regular schedule for bowel movements

Maintaining a regular schedule for bowel movements is essential for a healthy gut microbiome. Having consistent and timely elimination can prevent issues like constipation or diarrhea and support a balanced gut environment.

To establish a regular schedule:

- Listen to your body's natural cues and allocate time each day for a bowel movement.
- Find a time that works best for you, such as after a meal or in the morning, and make it a priority to visit the bathroom during that time.
- Create a relaxed environment, practice deep breathing, and avoid distractions to promote efficient elimination and a healthier gut.

Pay attention to your posture while using the toilet

The posture you adopt while using the toilet can significantly impact your gut health. The conventional sitting position on a toilet can restrict the natural flow of waste, potentially leading to issues like constipation or incomplete elimination.

To promote better gut health;

- Consider using a squatting position on the toilet.

You can achieve this by placing a small footstool or using specialized products that elevate your feet, allowing your knees to be higher than your hips.
This posture aligns the rectum and colon, facilitating easier elimination and reducing the risk of straining or constipation. Gradually incorporate this practice into your routine to improve your gut health and overall well-being.

Kick the habit of smoking

Smoking has detrimental effects on your gut microbiome and overall health. The chemicals present in cigarettes can disrupt the balance of gut bacteria, contribute to inflammation, and increase the risk of digestive disorders.

Quitting smoking is the best course of action to improve your gut health. Seek support from healthcare professionals, utilize nicotine replacement therapies if needed, and consider joining smoking cessation programs or support groups.

By quitting smoking, you can support a healthier gut microbiome, reduce inflammation, and lower the risk of associated health complications.

Dispose of processed foods

Transforming your gut microbiome and improving your health begins with eliminating processed foods from your diet. These convenience items are often laden with additives, preservatives, and unhealthy fats that wreak havoc on your gut bacteria.

By saying goodbye to processed foods, you pave the way for a healthier gut ecosystem.

How can you achieve this?

- Start by cleaning out your pantry and refrigerator.

Read labels carefully and avoid products with long lists of unrecognizable ingredients. Instead, focus on whole, unprocessed foods like fruits, vegetables, lean proteins, and whole grains. Your gut will thank you for this positive change.

#27

Fill up on fiber

Fiber is a crucial component in your journey to a transformed gut microbiome and improved health. It acts as a prebiotic, nourishing the beneficial bacteria in your gut. By increasing your fiber intake, you create an environment that supports the growth of these beneficial microbes.

Achieving this is simple:

- Incorporate fiber-rich foods into your meals. Enjoy a colorful assortment of fruits and vegetables, whole grains, legumes, and nuts.

These dietary additions not only promote a diverse and flourishing gut microbiome but also aid in digestion and provide a feeling of fullness, contributing to a healthier you.

Increase fiber for double the benefits

Boosting your fiber intake offers double the benefits for your gut microbiome and overall health. Not only does fiber provide nourishment for your beneficial gut bacteria, but it also helps regulate your bowel movements and supports healthy digestion.

To achieve this:

- Aim to gradually increase your daily fiber intake. Start by incorporating high-fiber foods such as chia seeds, flaxseeds, avocados, and bran cereals into your diet.

Remember to drink plenty of water to aid in the proper digestion of fiber. Embracing fiber-rich foods will not only improve your gut health but also enhance your overall well-being.

#29

Feast on fermented foods

One delicious way to transform your gut microbiome and improve your health is by indulging in fermented foods. These culinary delights are teeming with beneficial bacteria that can populate your gut and promote a thriving microbial community.

Achieving this is as simple as adding fermented foods to your meals. Include options like sauerkraut, kimchi, kefir, yogurt, and kombucha in your diet.

These probiotic powerhouses provide a range of health benefits, from enhanced digestion to strengthened immunity. So, savor the tangy goodness of fermented foods and let your gut flourish with each delectable bite.

#30

Enhance prebiotic intake

Nourishing your gut microbiome and optimizing your health can be achieved by enhancing your prebiotic intake. Prebiotics are a type of dietary fiber that serve as fuel for beneficial gut bacteria.

By consuming prebiotic-rich foods, you provide sustenance for these friendly microbes, allowing them to thrive and support your well-being. How can you achieve this? Incorporate foods like garlic, onions, leeks, asparagus, bananas, and oats into your daily meals.

These natural prebiotic sources will not only nourish your gut microbiome but also contribute to improved digestion and overall vitality.

Swap coffee for chicory root

If you're looking to transform your gut microbiome and enhance your health, consider swapping your daily cup of coffee for chicory root. While coffee can have some benefits, excessive consumption may negatively impact your gut bacteria.

In contrast, chicory root acts as a prebiotic, stimulating the growth of beneficial gut microbes. Achieving this switch is as simple as replacing your coffee with a chicory root-based herbal coffee alternative.

This change not only supports your gut health but may also lead to reduced caffeine intake and a smoother, more balanced energy throughout the day.

#32

Drink mushroom-infused beverages

Introducing mushroom-infused beverages into your routine can be a powerful step towards transforming your gut microbiome and improving your health. Certain mushrooms, such as reishi, lion's mane, and chaga, possess potent medicinal properties that positively influence gut health.

Achieving this change is as easy as:

- Incorporating mushroom teas or elixirs into your daily routine. These beverages provide a natural source of antioxidants, fiber, and beneficial compounds that promote a healthy gut microbiome.

So, sip on these earthy concoctions and let the magic of mushrooms work its wonders within you.

#33

Sip on black tea

While black tea is often enjoyed for its rich flavor, it can also contribute to a transformed gut microbiome and improved health. Black tea contains compounds called polyphenols, which act as prebiotics, nourishing your beneficial gut bacteria.

To achieve this:

- Simply replace some of your daily beverages with a cup of black tea. Whether you enjoy it hot or iced, with or without a splash of lemon, black tea can support the growth of a diverse and thriving gut microbiome.

So, sit back, relax, and sip your way to a healthier you.

Eliminate sugar

To transform your gut microbiome and improve your health, it's essential to eliminate or significantly reduce your sugar intake. Excessive sugar consumption can disrupt the balance of your gut bacteria, leading to inflammation and various health issues.

Achieving this change requires mindful choices;

- Start by cutting back on sugary beverages, processed snacks, and desserts. Instead, satisfy your sweet tooth with natural alternatives like fresh fruits or a small amount of honey.

By reducing sugar, you create an environment in your gut that supports the growth of beneficial bacteria, promoting overall well-being.

Avoid artificial sweeteners

While artificial sweeteners may seem like a tempting alternative to sugar, they can negatively impact your gut microbiome and compromise your health. Artificial sweeteners are associated with altered gut bacteria composition and increased risk of metabolic disorders.

Achieving this change involves reading labels and avoiding products that contain artificial sweeteners such as aspartame, sucralose, and saccharin. Instead, opt for natural sweeteners like stevia or small amounts of sugar if needed.

By avoiding artificial sweeteners, you support the balance and diversity of your gut microbiome, paving the way for improved health.

#36

Harness the power of quercetin

Unlocking the power of quercetin can be a game-changer in transforming your gut microbiome and improving your health. Quercetin is a flavonoid found in various fruits, vegetables, and herbs, known for its potent antioxidant and anti-inflammatory properties.

Achieving this transformation involves:

- Incorporating quercetin-rich foods into your diet.
- Indulge in the vibrant hues of berries, apples, onions, kale, and green tea.

These wholesome choices not only nourish your gut but also combat oxidative stress and inflammation, supporting your overall well-being.

So, embrace the beauty of quercetin-rich foods and let their healing touch ignite a positive change within you.

#37

Enjoy mango as a snack

Adding the luscious sweetness of mango to your snack repertoire can contribute to a transformed gut microbiome and improved health. Bursting with fiber, vitamins, and beneficial plant compounds, mangoes provide a tropical delight for your taste buds and your gut.

Achieving this is as simple as:

- Indulging in fresh mango slices as a snack or incorporating them into smoothies, salads, or salsas.

With each juicy bite, you nourish your body, support digestion, and delight in the flavors of nature's bounty.

So, let the vibrant allure of mango transport you to a healthier and more vibrant version of yourself.

#38

opt for slightly green bananas

Choosing slightly green bananas over fully ripe ones can be a small yet impactful step towards transforming your gut microbiome and enhancing your health. Unripe bananas contain resistant starch, a type of fiber that acts as a prebiotic, fueling the growth of beneficial gut bacteria.

Achieving this change involves:

- Selecting bananas with a hint of green and allowing them to ripen at home. Enjoy them sliced over yogurt, blended into smoothies, or baked into nutritious treats.

By opting for slightly green bananas, you provide nourishment to your gut and set the stage for a thriving microbial community, fostering a healthier you.

Reintroduce white potatoes

Reintroducing white potatoes into your diet can be a comforting and beneficial move for your gut microbiome and overall health. While often misunderstood, white potatoes are a good source of resistant starch, a prebiotic fiber that supports the growth of beneficial gut bacteria.

Achieving this reintroduction is as easy as including:

- Boiled or roasted white potatoes in your meals. Enjoy them as a side dish or incorporate them into hearty salads.

By embracing the humble white potato, you provide your gut with nourishment and create an environment that promotes optimal digestion and well-being.

Cook and cool starches

Transforming your gut microbiome and optimizing your health can be as simple as changing the way you prepare starches. Cooking and cooling starchy foods like potatoes, rice, and pasta can enhance their resistant starch content. Resistant starch acts as a prebiotic, fueling the growth of beneficial gut bacteria.

To achieve this:

- Cook your starches as usual and then allow them to cool before consuming.

This change in preparation method not only adds versatility to your meals but also supports a thriving gut microbiome, leading to improved digestion and overall vitality.

Cleanse and purify the air around you

The air quality in your surroundings can influence your gut microbiome and overall health. Pollutants, allergens, and mold in the air can have detrimental effects on gut bacteria and contribute to various health issues.

To improve air quality:

- Ensure proper ventilation in your living spaces, regularly clean and dust your environment, and
- Consider using air purifiers or natural air-filtering plants.

Minimize the use of harsh chemical cleaners and opt for natural alternatives to prevent the release of harmful substances into the air you breathe.

By purifying the air around you, you can create a healthier environment for your gut microbiome to thrive.

#42

Establish a daily routine

Establishing a daily routine can have a positive impact on your gut microbiome and overall health. Consistency in meal times, sleep schedules, exercise routines, and relaxation practices helps synchronize your body's natural circadian rhythm, which plays a vital role in digestion, metabolism, and gut microbial balance.

Prioritize self-care, stress management, and healthy habits within your daily routine. Set specific times for meals, allocate time for exercise, ensure adequate sleep, and incorporate relaxation techniques such as meditation or deep breathing.

By maintaining a daily routine, you support a harmonious gut microbiome and overall well-being.

Get rid of antacids

Antacids, often used to manage heartburn or acid reflux, can disrupt the balance of your gut microbiome. These medications reduce stomach acid, which is essential for proper digestion and maintaining a healthy gut environment.

Instead of relying on antacids, consider identifying and addressing the root causes of your digestive issues. Adopt lifestyle changes such as eating smaller, more frequent meals, avoiding trigger foods, managing stress, and maintaining a healthy weight.

These measures can help alleviate symptoms naturally, restore gut health, and promote a balanced gut microbiome.

#44

Limit your alcohol consumption

Excessive alcohol consumption can harm the delicate balance of your gut microbiome and contribute to digestive disorders. Alcohol can increase intestinal permeability (leaky gut), disrupt microbial diversity, and promote inflammation in the gut.

To support a healthier gut microbiome:

- It is crucial to limit your alcohol intake.
- Adhere to recommended guidelines for moderate drinking, which typically means up to one drink per day for women and up to two drinks per day for men.
- Alternatively, consider abstaining from alcohol entirely to promote a healthier gut microbiome and overall well-being.

It is important to note that individual experiences may vary, and it's always recommended to consult with healthcare professionals or registered dietitians for personalized advice and guidance on improving gut health.

#45

Manage your magnesium levels

Magnesium, often referred to as the relaxation mineral, plays a vital role in maintaining gut health. Adequate magnesium levels support proper digestion, promote regular bowel movements, and facilitate the growth of beneficial gut bacteria.

Embrace magnesium-rich foods, such as leafy greens, nuts, seeds, and whole grains, in your diet. Additionally, consider incorporating magnesium supplements under the guidance of a healthcare professional to ensure optimal levels.

By managing your magnesium intake, you provide a nurturing environment for your gut microbiome, fostering harmony and vitality within.

#46

Avoid exposure to heavy metals

Heavy metals, such as lead, mercury, and arsenic, can disrupt your gut microbiome and compromise your overall well-being. Take proactive steps to minimize exposure to these toxic substances in your environment.

Be mindful of contaminated water sources, choose organic produce when possible, and limit consumption of fish known to be high in mercury.

Additionally, consider implementing detoxification strategies, such as consuming foods rich in detoxifying agents or seeking professional guidance for chelation therapy. By reducing heavy metal exposure, you safeguard the delicate balance of your gut microbiome and protect your health.

Take steps to minimize high histamine levels

Histamine intolerance can wreak havoc on your gut health, leading to digestive disturbances, inflammation, and discomfort. Be aware of foods and environmental factors that contribute to high histamine levels.

Limit your intake of histamine-rich foods, such as fermented foods, aged cheeses, and cured meats. Additionally, consider incorporating natural antihistamines, such as quercetin or vitamin C, into your routine.

Working with a healthcare professional well-versed in histamine intolerance can help you navigate this complex condition and restore balance to your gut microbiome.

#48

Seek a thorough evaluation of your thyroid

Your thyroid health profoundly influences your gut microbiome and overall well-being. If you experience symptoms of thyroid dysfunction, such as fatigue, weight changes, or mood disturbances, seek a comprehensive evaluation from a healthcare professional.

Thyroid imbalances can disrupt the delicate equilibrium of your gut microbiome, leading to digestive issues and compromised immune function. Collaborate with your healthcare provider to assess thyroid hormone levels, explore potential underlying causes, and develop an integrative treatment plan.

By optimizing your thyroid health, you lay a solid foundation for a flourishing gut microbiome and vibrant vitality.

#49

Pinch your arm to assess your body's response

Take a moment to connect with your physical self and gently pinch your arm. Notice how your body responds to this simple act.

Does it feel resilient and strong, or do you experience discomfort or tenderness? Pay attention to any sensations or changes in your body. This small gesture serves as a reminder of the interconnectedness between your gut health and overall well-being.

#50

Take a breath and undergo a test

Deep breath in, deep breath out. Inhale the possibility of better health and exhale any doubts or fears. Consider undergoing diagnostic tests or assessments to gain deeper insights into your gut microbiome and overall health.

Whether it's a stool analysis, breath test, or other specialized examinations, these tests can provide valuable information about the state of your gut.

Embrace the opportunity to learn more about your body, empowering yourself with knowledge and paving the way for targeted interventions and personalized healing.

#51

Analyze and manage your stress levels closely

Stress, both internal and external, can take a toll on your gut health. Reflect on your daily life and identify sources of stress that may be impacting your well-being.

Are there work pressures, relationship challenges, or self-imposed expectations that contribute to your stress? Take proactive steps to manage and mitigate stress through practices such as meditation, yoga, or engaging in activities that bring you joy.

By prioritizing stress management, you create a nurturing environment for your gut microbiome to thrive. Nurture your emotional well-being, and let the resilience of your gut mirror the strength within your soul.

#52

Examine your skin for any abnormalities

Your skin is an external reflection of your internal health, including your gut microbiome. Take the time to scrutinize your skin, noticing any changes, blemishes, or abnormalities that may be present.

Is your skin glowing and vibrant, or do you notice signs of inflammation or imbalance? If you have concerns, consult with a dermatologist or healthcare professional to address any underlying issues.

Nourish your skin from the inside out by providing your gut microbiome with the support it needs to promote healthy skin and radiance.

#53

Ponder upon your regularity of bowel movements

The rhythm and regularity of your bowel movements can provide valuable insights into your gut health. Take a moment to contemplate your current pattern of elimination.

Do you experience regular and effortless bowel movements, or are there irregularities or discomfort? Strive for consistency and establish healthy habits that promote regularity, such as staying hydrated, consuming fiber-rich foods, and maintaining a balanced lifestyle.

Your gut health relies on the smooth functioning of your digestive system, and fostering a harmonious relationship with your bowel movements cultivates a sense of balance and well-being.

Control your cravings for sugar

Sugar cravings can sabotage your gut health and overall well-being. Reflect on your relationship with sugar and observe the patterns and triggers that lead to cravings.

Are you reaching for sugary treats in times of stress or emotional turmoil? Take charge of your cravings by adopting a whole-food, nutrient-dense diet that supports your gut microbiome and stabilizes your blood sugar levels.

Embrace the sweetness of nourishing fruits and natural alternatives like stevia or monk fruit to satisfy your taste buds without compromising your gut health.

#55

Consult the scale to track your progress

While weight is not the sole indicator of health, monitoring your progress can provide insights into your overall well-being. Step onto the scale and consider the numbers as part of the bigger picture.

Celebrate any positive changes, whether they are physical, emotional, or mental. Remember that your gut health journey is about nourishing and healing your body from the inside out, and the scale can be a tool to gauge your progress, but not the sole measure of your success.

#56

Keep a log of your headaches

Headaches can be indicators of underlying imbalances in your gut microbiome. Maintain a journal to document the frequency, intensity, and potential triggers of your headaches.

By identifying patterns and potential associations with certain foods, stressors, or environmental factors, you can make informed decisions to support your gut health.

Consult with healthcare professionals to explore potential solutions and find relief from headaches, unlocking a renewed sense of vitality and well-being.

Check for any bloating or discomfort

Bloating and discomfort can be signs of gut imbalance. Take a moment to assess your body and notice any sensations of bloating, distention, or discomfort in your abdomen.

If you experience these symptoms regularly, consult with a healthcare professional to investigate potential underlying causes and develop a personalized plan to address them.

Embrace the opportunity to restore harmony within your gut, bidding farewell to discomfort and welcoming a renewed sense of ease and lightness.

#58

Be mindful of any fluctuations in your mood

Your gut and brain are intimately connected through the gut-brain axis, influencing your mood and emotional well-being. Reflect on your emotional landscape and notice any fluctuations or imbalances in your mood.

Are you experiencing heightened anxiety, low mood, or irritability? Nurture your gut microbiome through the transformative solutions discussed earlier, as they can play a significant role in promoting emotional balance and fostering a positive outlook on life.

#59

Stay vigilant for any signs

By staying aware and attentive to the subtle cues and signals your body sends, you can proactively identify potential issues with your gut microbiome. These signs may include changes in bowel movements, digestive discomfort, or irregularities in your overall well-being. Paying close attention to these signs empowers you to take timely action and nurture a healthier gut.

To achieve this:

- Practice mindfulness and self-awareness.
- Cultivate a deep connection with your body, listening to its whispers and acknowledging any shifts in your physical and emotional state.
- Keep a keen eye on any changes that may indicate an imbalance in your gut microbiome.

#60

Document your experiences in a journal

Maintaining a journal is an invaluable tool in your journey towards transforming your gut microbiome and improving your health. It allows you to track patterns, identify triggers, and make informed decisions about your diet and lifestyle.

Create a dedicated journal to record your daily experiences, including your meals, emotions, stress levels, and any symptoms you may encounter. By documenting this information, you can establish connections between your gut health and various factors that influence it.

This awareness empowers you to make targeted changes and assess the effectiveness of different interventions.

Remove certain foods from your diet

Your dietary choices have a profound impact on the composition and diversity of your gut microbiome. To foster a healthier gut, consider eliminating foods that may disrupt its balance. These may include processed foods, refined sugars, artificial additives, and excessive consumption of certain fats.

Begin by gradually removing these culprits from your diet, replacing them with whole, nutrient-dense foods. Embrace a plant-based diet rich in fiber, vibrant fruits and vegetables, and wholesome grains.

This transition provides nourishment to beneficial gut bacteria while depriving harmful microbes of their preferred fuel.

Prioritize observing before you flush

Your daily trip to the bathroom offers a valuable opportunity to gather insights into your gut health. Before flushing, take a moment to observe the characteristics of your stool. Pay attention to its consistency, color, and any unusual features.

Healthy bowel movements are typically well-formed, easy to pass, and exhibit a medium-brown color. Deviations from this norm may indicate imbalances or potential digestive issues.

By prioritizing this observation, you can catch early warning signs and make adjustments to your diet or seek appropriate medical guidance if necessary.

#63

Be aware of any floaters you may encounter

Floating stools can be a potential indicator of malabsorption or imbalances within your gut. When you notice these floaters, it's essential to acknowledge their presence and investigate further.

Consider consulting with a healthcare professional who specializes in gut health. They can help identify the underlying causes and develop a tailored plan to restore balance within your gut microbiome.

Through their guidance, you can regain control over your digestive well-being and experience improved overall health.

Take a moment to sense the aroma

The aroma of your breath, sweat, and bodily secretions can provide valuable clues about your gut health. Unpleasant odors may indicate imbalances or metabolic issues that need attention.

Take a moment to breathe in deeply and sense these aromas. If you notice persistent or unusual smells, it's wise to seek professional guidance.

A healthcare provider can conduct thorough assessments and recommend appropriate interventions to address the root causes, helping you achieve a healthier gut and a renewed sense of freshness.

#65

Show concern for the color you see

The color of your urine and other bodily fluids can serve as an indicator of your internal well-being. While shades may vary due to factors like hydration and diet, it's crucial to pay attention to any significant deviations from the norm.

If you consistently observe unusual colors, such as dark yellow or reddish tinges, it's advisable to consult a healthcare professional.

They can evaluate potential underlying conditions, assess your gut health, and guide you towards implementing changes that restore balance and vibrant health.

#66

Set a timer to stay on track

Establishing regular meal times and sticking to them can have a positive impact on your gut microbiome. By setting a timer or creating a meal schedule, you cultivate a rhythm that supports optimal digestion and absorption of nutrients.

Consistency in meal timing promotes a healthy circadian rhythm, which influences your gut microbiome's composition and function. Aim for balanced meals containing a variety of whole foods, and avoid rushing through your meals.

This intentional approach fosters a harmonious relationship with your gut, ensuring it receives the nourishment it needs to thrive.

#67

Embrace the Art of Home Cooking

Embracing home cooking can have a transformative effect on your gut microbiome and overall health. By preparing meals at home, you have control over the ingredients and cooking methods, allowing you to prioritize nutrient-dense, whole foods. This helps promote a diverse and balanced gut microbiome.

To achieve this, start by;

- Planning your meals in advance, incorporating a variety of fruits, vegetables, whole grains, and lean proteins.
- Avoid processed foods high in artificial additives and unhealthy fats.
- Experiment with different cooking techniques like steaming, sautéing, or baking to retain nutrients.
- Gradually reduce your reliance on pre-packaged meals and opt for homemade alternatives. With time, your gut microbiome will benefit from the nourishing and wholesome meals you create.

#68

Dissolve and Disrupt Biofilms

Biofilms are communities of microorganisms that form on surfaces, including the lining of your gut. Disrupting biofilms can help improve gut health by preventing harmful bacteria from thriving and potentially causing inflammation.

Achieving this involves:

- Incorporating natural biofilm disruptors into your routine. These include certain enzymes like serrapeptase or nattokinase, which can help dissolve biofilms. You can find these enzymes in supplement form.

Additionally;

- Consuming foods rich in polyphenols, such as cranberries, green tea, and garlic, can also assist in biofilm disruption.

Regularly including these biofilm disruptors in your diet can contribute to a healthier gut microbiome.

#69

Explore the Benefits of Colostrum

Colostrum, the nutrient-rich milk produced by mammals shortly after giving birth, offers numerous benefits for gut health. It contains bioactive compounds, growth factors, and immunoglobulins that can support a healthy gut microbiome.

To explore the benefits of colostrum, consider incorporating colostrum supplements into your daily routine. Look for high-quality, pure colostrum sourced from reputable producers. Start with a recommended dosage and gradually increase as needed.

Colostrum can help modulate the gut microbiome, improve gut barrier function, and promote a balanced immune response, leading to enhanced overall health.

#70

Cleanse Your System from Parasites

Parasites can disrupt the delicate balance of the gut microbiome and negatively impact your health. Cleansing your system from parasites can help restore harmony in your gut and improve overall well-being.

To achieve this, consult with a healthcare professional to determine the most appropriate parasite cleanse protocol for you. This may involve herbal supplements known to have anti-parasitic properties, such as black walnut, wormwood, and cloves. Follow the recommended dosage and duration as directed by your healthcare provider.

Additionally, practice good hygiene, wash your hands regularly, and ensure proper food handling to minimize the risk of reinfection.

Restore the Health of Your Gut

Restoring the health of your gut is essential for overall well-being. A healthy gut microbiome promotes efficient digestion, absorption of nutrients, and supports a robust immune system.

To restore your gut health, start by;

- Incorporating fermented foods into your diet. These include yogurt, kefir, sauerkraut, and kimchi, which provide beneficial bacteria for your gut.
- Consider taking a high-quality probiotic supplement to further support microbial balance.
- Reduce your intake of processed foods, refined sugars, and artificial additives, as they can disrupt the gut microbiome. Instead, focus on consuming a wide variety of fiber-rich foods, such as fruits, vegetables, legumes, and whole grains, to nourish your gut bacteria.

Consulting with a healthcare professional or registered dietitian can provide personalized guidance tailored to your specific needs.

#72

Embrace Daily Digestive Regularity

Establishing daily digestive regularity is crucial for maintaining a healthy gut microbiome. Regular bowel movements help eliminate waste, prevent constipation, and support the growth of beneficial bacteria.

To achieve daily digestive regularity:

- Prioritize hydration by drinking an adequate amount of water throughout the day.
- Increase your fiber intake gradually by consuming fruits, vegetables, whole grains, and legumes. These fiber-rich foods promote regular bowel movements and feed the beneficial bacteria in your gut.
- Engage in regular physical activity to stimulate bowel movements.

Additionally, establish a consistent daily routine for meals and bathroom visits to help regulate your digestive system. If you experience persistent digestive issues, consult with a healthcare professional for further evaluation and guidance.

#73

Bounce and Rejuvenate on a Trampoline

Engaging in trampoline exercises can provide numerous benefits for your gut microbiome and overall health. The bouncing motion stimulates lymphatic circulation, which helps remove toxins from the body and supports a healthy immune system.

Regular trampoline workouts can also improve digestion and contribute to a balanced gut microbiome.

To achieve this;

- Consider purchasing a mini-trampoline or visiting a trampoline park. Start with gentle bouncing and gradually increase intensity and duration as your fitness level improves.

Aim for regular sessions of trampoline exercise, allowing your body to rejuvenate and reap the benefits of improved gut health.

Indulge in the Relaxation of a Lymphatic Massage

A lymphatic massage is a gentle, therapeutic massage technique that can benefit the gut microbiome and overall well-being. It helps stimulate lymphatic circulation, facilitating the removal of waste and toxins from the body.

By supporting lymphatic drainage, a massage can promote a healthier gut environment.

To experience the benefits of a lymphatic massage;

- Seek out a licensed massage therapist with expertise in lymphatic drainage techniques. During the massage, gentle pressure is applied to specific areas of the body to encourage lymphatic flow.

Regular sessions can help enhance gut health and improve overall lymphatic function.

Give Your Oral Health the Attention It Deserves

Oral health plays a crucial role in maintaining a healthy gut microbiome. The mouth is the entry point for food and bacteria, and an imbalance of oral bacteria can impact the gut ecosystem.

To give your oral health the attention it deserves, Establish a consistent oral hygiene routine.

- Brush your teeth twice a day with a fluoride toothpaste and use dental floss or interdental brushes to clean between teeth.
- Consider incorporating a tongue scraper to remove bacteria from the tongue surface.
- Regular dental check-ups and professional cleanings are also essential to address any oral health issues.

By maintaining good oral hygiene practices, you can support a healthier gut microbiome.

#76

Embrace Natural Oral Care— Ditch the Mouthwash

As part of your oral care routine, consider embracing natural alternatives to conventional mouthwash. Traditional mouthwashes often contain alcohol and other harsh ingredients that can disrupt the oral microbiome.

To achieve this;

- Explore natural oral care options such as oil pulling. This involves swishing a tablespoon of coconut oil or sesame oil in your mouth for 10-15 minutes, then spitting it out.
- Oil pulling can help reduce harmful bacteria in the mouth without disturbing the beneficial oral microbiome.

Additionally, herbal mouth rinses made with santimicrobial herbs like tea tree oil or peppermint can provide a refreshing alternative.

Consult with a dental professional for personalized recommendations based on your oral health needs.

Prioritize Physical Activity and Move More

Regular physical activity is essential for maintaining a healthy gut microbiome and overall health. Exercise helps stimulate bowel movements, supports a diverse gut microbiome, and promotes overall well-being.

To prioritize physical activity;

- Find activities you enjoy and incorporate them into your routine.
- Aim for at least 150 minutes of moderate-intensity aerobic exercise or 75 minutes of vigorous-intensity exercise each week, as recommended by health guidelines. This can include brisk walking, jogging, cycling, swimming, or engaging in sports or fitness classes.

Additionally, incorporate strength training exercises to build muscle and support a healthy metabolism. By making physical activity a priority, you can positively impact your gut microbiome and enhance your overall health.

#78

Upgrade Your Sleeping Sanctuary with a New Bed

Sleep plays a vital role in maintaining a healthy gut microbiome. Upgrading your sleeping environment, particularly your bed, can contribute to better sleep quality and overall well-being.

To achieve this;

- Consider investing in a new mattress and pillows that provide proper support and comfort.
- Look for options that align with your preferred sleeping position and provide adequate spinal alignment.

Additionally, choose bedding made from natural and breathable materials to promote a comfortable sleep environment. Establish a consistent sleep schedule and create a relaxing bedtime routine to optimize your sleep hygiene.

By prioritizing quality sleep, you support a healthy gut microbiome and improve your overall health.

#79

Opt for Alternatives to Antibiotics

While antibiotics have their place in medical treatment, excessive and unnecessary use can disrupt the gut microbiome. Opting for alternatives to antibiotics whenever possible can help preserve the balance of beneficial bacteria in your gut.

To achieve this;

- Consult with your healthcare provider to explore non-antibiotic options for managing infections or illnesses.
- In some cases, natural remedies, supportive therapies, or targeted treatments may be suitable alternatives.

However, always follow the guidance of your healthcare professional to ensure proper management of your health condition.

By using antibiotics judiciously and considering alternative approaches, you can help maintain a healthy gut microbiome.

#80

Alleviate Heartburn by Drinking the Right Remedies

Heartburn and acid reflux can disrupt the gut microbiome and cause discomfort. Drinking the right remedies can help alleviate these symptoms and promote a healthier digestive system.

To achieve relief:

- Consider sipping on natural remedies that help soothe heartburn, such as ginger tea, chamomile tea, or aloe vera juice. These beverages can help reduce inflammation and provide a calming effect on the digestive system.

Additionally, avoid trigger foods that may exacerbate heartburn, such as spicy or fatty foods, caffeine, and citrus fruits. Adopting a mindful eating approach and eating smaller, more frequent meals can also contribute to better digestion and reduced heartburn symptoms.

Consult with a healthcare professional if heartburn persists or becomes chronic.

#81

Soothe Your Senses with a Cup of Peppermint Tea

Peppermint tea offers several benefits for the gut microbiome and digestive health. It contains compounds like menthol that have a calming effect on the digestive system and can alleviate symptoms such as bloating and indigestion.

To experience the benefits of peppermint tea;

- Steep a peppermint tea bag in hot water for 5-10 minutes and enjoy it after meals or when experiencing digestive discomfort. Be mindful of any potential sensitivities or interactions with existing health conditions or medications.

Peppermint tea can serve as a soothing and refreshing addition to your daily routine, promoting a healthier gut microbiome.

#82

Experience the Benefits of Needle Therapy

Needle therapy, also known as acupuncture, can contribute to improved gut health by promoting better digestion and balancing the body's energy flow. It involves the insertion of thin needles into specific points on the body, stimulating the body's natural healing processes.

To experience the benefits of needle therapy;

- Seek a qualified acupuncturist with experience in gastrointestinal health. During a session, the acupuncturist will assess your specific needs and target specific acupuncture points to support gut health.

This therapy can help regulate digestive function, reduce inflammation, and promote a healthier gut microbiome. Regular sessions may be necessary to achieve optimal results.

#83

Boost Your Glutathione Levels for Overall Well-being

Glutathione is a powerful antioxidant that plays a crucial role in maintaining a healthy gut microbiome and overall well-being. It helps protect the gut lining, supports detoxification, and supports a balanced immune response.

To boost glutathione levels;

- Focus on lifestyle factors that support its production. These include consuming foods rich in glutathione precursors, such as cruciferous vegetables (broccoli, cauliflower), asparagus, and avocado.

Additionally, certain supplements like N-acetylcysteine (NAC), alpha-lipoic acid (ALA), and milk thistle can help support glutathione production.

Prioritize a well-rounded diet, exercise regularly, manage stress levels, and avoid exposure to toxins to optimize glutathione levels naturally.

Nourish and Support Your Liver's Vital Functions

The health of your liver is closely connected to the gut microbiome. Nourishing and supporting the liver's vital functions can have a positive impact on gut health and overall well-being.

To achieve this;

- Focus on consuming liver-supportive foods and herbs. These include cruciferous vegetables, leafy greens, garlic, turmeric, and dandelion root. These foods contain compounds that aid in liver detoxification and promote a healthy gut microbiome.
- Avoid excessive alcohol consumption, as it can harm the liver and disrupt gut health.
- Stay hydrated, exercise regularly, and maintain a healthy weight to support optimal liver function.

If you have underlying liver conditions, consult with a healthcare professional for personalized guidance.

Rejuvenate Your Skin with Gentle Brushing

Dry brushing is a practice that involves using a natural bristle brush to gently exfoliate the skin. This technique can stimulate lymphatic circulation and contribute to a healthier gut microbiome.

To rejuvenate your skin with gentle brushing;

- Use a dry brush with natural bristles and perform the brushing before showering. Start from your feet and move upward, using gentle, upward strokes.
- Avoid sensitive areas or broken skin. Dry brushing can help remove dead skin cells, enhance blood flow, and support lymphatic drainage, which indirectly benefits the gut microbiome.

Incorporate dry brushing into your self-care routine a few times a week for optimal results.

#86

Embrace an Environmentally Friendly Lifestyle

Adopting an environmentally friendly lifestyle not only benefits the planet but also has a positive impact on your gut microbiome and overall health. Making conscious choices to reduce exposure to harmful chemicals and pollutants can support a balanced gut ecosystem.

To embrace an environmentally friendly lifestyle:

- Prioritize organic and locally sourced foods whenever possible.
- Reduce the use of plastic and opt for reusable or sustainable alternatives.
- Choose natural cleaning products that are free from harsh chemicals to minimize their impact on your gut microbiome.
- Practice mindful consumption, recycling, and waste reduction to contribute to a healthier environment and, consequently, a healthier gut microbiome.

#87

Cleanse and Renew Your Gut Health

Periodic gut cleansing can help eliminate toxins, support a balanced gut microbiome, and improve overall health. Cleansing protocols can involve various approaches, such as dietary modifications, fasting, or specific cleansing supplements.

To cleanse and renew your gut health:

- Consider consulting with a healthcare professional or registered dietitian experienced in gut health. They can guide you through an appropriate cleansing protocol based on your specific needs and health status.
- Engaging in a gentle cleanse for a designated period can help eliminate harmful substances and reset your gut microbiome.

Follow the recommended guidelines, maintain hydration, and prioritize nutrient-dense foods to support the cleansing process effectively.

Stimulate and Massage Your Bowels

Stimulating and massaging your bowels can support regular bowel movements, promote healthy digestion, and contribute to a balanced gut microbiome.

To stimulate and massage your bowels;

- Consider incorporating techniques such as abdominal self-massage or acupressure. With clean hands, apply gentle pressure to the abdomen in a circular motion, following the path of the colon.
- Engaging in regular physical activity, such as walking or yoga, can also stimulate bowel movements.
- Practicing deep breathing exercises can help relax the digestive system and promote bowel regularity.

If you experience chronic constipation or digestive issues, consult with a healthcare professional for personalized guidance.

Take Your Exercise Routine Outdoors

Exercising outdoors provides additional benefits for the gut microbiome and overall health. Outdoor exercise exposes you to natural environments and fresh air, which can positively impact gut health and well-being.

To take your exercise routine outdoors:

- Explore outdoor activities such as walking, jogging, cycling, hiking, or practicing yoga in nature.
- Engaging in outdoor activities not only supports physical fitness but also allows you to connect with nature and reduce stress levels.
- Spending time in green spaces has been linked to improved mood, reduced inflammation, and enhanced gut health.
- Incorporate outdoor workouts into your routine to promote a healthier gut microbiome.

#90

Fuel Your Body with Glutamine for Optimal Performance

Glutamine is an amino acid that plays a crucial role in gut health and overall well-being. It supports the integrity of the gut lining and promotes the growth of beneficial bacteria.

To fuel your body with glutamine:

- Focus on consuming foods rich in this amino acid. Good dietary sources include beef, poultry, fish, dairy products, tofu, legumes, and leafy greens.

Additionally, you can consider glutamine supplements under the guidance of a healthcare professional, especially if you have specific health conditions.

By providing your body with adequate glutamine, you support a healthy gut microbiome and promote optimal performance.

Take a peek at your urine

Monitoring the color and clarity of your urine provides insights into your hydration status and overall gut health. Adequate hydration is crucial for maintaining optimal digestive function and supporting a diverse gut microbiome.

Take a moment to observe the color of your urine. Ideally, it should be pale yellow or straw-colored, indicating proper hydration. Darker shades may suggest dehydration, while excessively light or clear urine might signify overhydration.

Strive for a healthy balance by drinking enough water throughout the day, adjusting intake based on activity levels and environmental factors.

Maintain a journal of your bowel movements

Regular bowel movements are essential for a healthy gut and overall well-being. By keeping a bowel movement journal, you can track frequency, consistency, and any associated symptoms.

Make a habit of recording details such as time of day, stool consistency, and any changes you notice. This journal can serve as a valuable resource when discussing your gut health with a healthcare professional.

It enables them to assess patterns and make targeted recommendations to improve your gut microbiome, leading to enhanced digestive function and improved health.

#93

Take a whiff of your breath

Your breath holds secrets that can unlock the mysteries of your gut health. As you exhale, take a moment to notice any unusual or unpleasant odors lingering in the air. Foul breath can be an indication of imbalances within your gut microbiome.

Don't be disheartened if you detect an unwelcome scent. Instead, let it be a gentle reminder to prioritize your gut health.

Seek the guidance of a healthcare professional who can delve deeper into the root causes and offer personalized strategies to freshen your breath and restore harmony within your gut.

#94

Give your underarms a sniff

Our bodies communicate with us through various channels, and our underarms are no exception. Take a moment to inhale and detect any unusual odors emanating from this area. Strong or unpleasant odors can signify imbalances in your gut microbiome.

Don't let embarrassment discourage you from taking action. Instead, embrace this opportunity to explore natural deodorant options and consider adjustments to your diet and lifestyle.

By addressing the underlying causes of body odor, you can create an environment where beneficial bacteria thrive, fostering a healthier gut and a newfound sense of confidence.

Pay close attention to the state of your tongue

Your tongue, with its unique texture and appearance, can provide valuable insights into your gut health. Take a moment to observe its color, coating, and any unusual changes. A white or yellowish coating may indicate imbalances in your gut microbiome.

Cultivate a habit of tongue scraping or gently brushing your tongue daily to maintain oral hygiene and promote a healthy oral microbiome.

Additionally, consult with a healthcare professional who can help you identify and address any underlying gut-related issues, leading to improved tongue health and overall well-being.

#96

Perform a spit test to assess your health

Surprisingly, a simple spit test can offer insights into the health of your gut microbiome. Upon waking up in the morning, gather some saliva in your mouth and observe its consistency and clarity. Excessive thickness or cloudiness may suggest imbalances in your gut.

If you notice any abnormalities, consider consulting a healthcare professional who specializes in gut health. They can guide you through personalized interventions, such as dietary modifications and targeted supplementation, to restore balance within your gut microbiome.

This proactive approach empowers you to reclaim your health and vitality.

#97

Give your digestive system a beet boost

Beets, with their vibrant colors and earthy flavors, offer a powerful ally in transforming your gut microbiome. These root vegetables contain beneficial compounds that support digestive health and promote a diverse microbial ecosystem.

Incorporate beets into your diet by enjoying them raw, juiced, roasted, or blended into smoothies. Their natural fiber content nourishes gut bacteria, while antioxidants and phytonutrients provide anti-inflammatory benefits.

Embrace the goodness of beets and witness the transformative effects on your gut health and overall vitality.

#98

Generate bubbles with some baking soda

Baking soda, a pantry staple, possesses remarkable properties that can help rebalance your gut microbiome. Mix a teaspoon of baking soda in a glass of water and observe the fizzing bubbles. This effervescence can signify adequate stomach acid levels, essential for optimal digestion.

If the bubbles are slow to appear or barely noticeable, it may indicate low stomach acid production.

Consider discussing this with a healthcare professional who can guide you through targeted interventions, such as betaine HCl supplementation or dietary adjustments, to improve digestion and restore gut health.

Feel the burning sensation of Betaine HCl

Betaine HCl, a natural compound found in the stomach, plays a vital role in breaking down food and maintaining a healthy gut environment. By supplementing with Betaine HCl under the guidance of a healthcare professional, you can assess your body's response.

Take note of any warm or burning sensation after consuming a Betaine HCl supplement. This sensation indicates that your stomach acid levels are being appropriately supported.

The therapeutic use of Betaine HCl can aid digestion, enhance nutrient absorption, and promote a balanced gut microbiome, contributing to your overall well-being.

#100

Determine if you have any sensitivities

Food sensitivities can wreak havoc on your gut health, leading to inflammation, discomfort, and imbalances in your microbiome. Pay close attention to how your body reacts to certain foods by keeping a detailed food diary.

Note any symptoms or changes you experience after consuming specific foods. This self-awareness empowers you to identify potential sensitivities or intolerances. Consider working with a healthcare professional or registered dietitian to conduct an elimination diet or food sensitivity testing.

By eliminating trigger foods and reintroducing them strategically, you can pinpoint the culprits and tailor your diet to support a thriving gut microbiome.

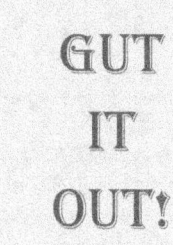

GUT
IT
OUT!

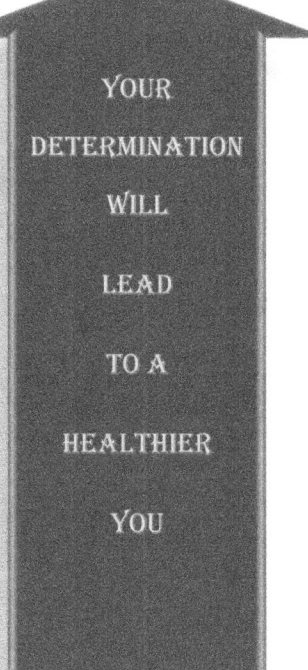

YOUR
DETERMINATION
WILL

LEAD

TO A

HEALTHIER

YOU